DYSLEXIA:
I LIVE WITH IT

Randymary de Rosier

BALBOA
PRESS
A DIVISION OF HAY HOUSE

Copyright © 2018 Randymary de Rosier.

All rights reserved. No part of this book may be used or reproduced by any means, graphic, electronic, or mechanical, including photocopying, recording, taping or by any information storage retrieval system without the written permission of the author except in the case of brief quotations embodied in critical articles and reviews.

Balboa Press books may be ordered through booksellers or by contacting:

Balboa Press
A Division of Hay House
1663 Liberty Drive
Bloomington, IN 47403
www.balboapress.com
1 (877) 407-4847

Because of the dynamic nature of the Internet, any web addresses or links contained in this book may have changed since publication and may no longer be valid. The views expressed in this work are solely those of the author and do not necessarily reflect the views of the publisher, and the publisher hereby disclaims any responsibility for them.

The author of this book does not dispense medical advice or prescribe the use of any technique as a form of treatment for physical, emotional, or medical problems without the advice of a physician, either directly or indirectly. The intent of the author is only to offer information of a general nature to help you in your quest for emotional and spiritual well-being. In the event you use any of the information in this book for yourself, which is your constitutional right, the author and the publisher assume no responsibility for your actions.

Any people depicted in stock imagery provided by Getty Images are models, and such images are being used for illustrative purposes only. Certain stock imagery © Getty Images.

Print information available on the last page.

ISBN: 978-1-9822-0587-4 (sc)
ISBN: 978-1-9822-0589-8 (hc)
ISBN: 978-1-9822-0588-1 (e)

Library of Congress Control Number: 2018906713

Balboa Press rev. date: 07/09/2018

CONTENTS

Acknowledgements ix
From The Author xi
Introduction xix

Chapter One:	Brain Malfunction Named 1
Chapter Two:	Family 3
Chapter Three:	School 11
Chapter Four:	"You Are Not College Material" 15
Chapter Five:	Venturing Out 21
Chapter Six:	Coping 25
Chapter Seven:	University 31
Chapter Eight:	Diagnosed To Get Help 37
Chapter Nine:	Finding My Voice 45
Chapter Ten:	Living Alone vs. Being Alone 51
Chapter eleven:	Butterfly 55
Chapter Twelve:	Learned Tricks and Techniques 59
Chapter Thirteen:	Inspiration 67
Chapter Fourteen:	Conclusion 73

Post Script 79

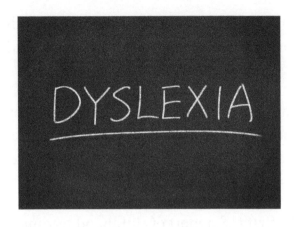

HISTORY OF DEVELOPMENTAL DYSLEXIA

Dyslexia was identified by Oswald Berkhan in 1881, but the term *dyslexia* was coined in 1887 by Rudolf Berlin, an ophthalmologist in Stuttgart. He used the term to refer to the case of a young boy who had a severe impairment in learning to read and write, despite showing typical intelligence and physical abilities in all other respects.

In 1896, W. Pringle Morgan, a British physician from Seaford, East Sussex, published a description of a reading-specific learning disorder in a report to the *British Medical Journal* titled "Congenital Word Blindness". performance. : From: Wikipedia, the free encyclopedia

'Learning disabilities' hasn't always been a household term. We only began to discover the reasons for learning problems a little over a century ago, and many people still have to fight for rights to equal opportunities and appropriate education.

This timeline tracks the history of learning disabilities, from their discovery in 1877 to our most recent laws and scientific findings.

1877 – The term "word blindness"; is coined by German neurologist Adolf Kussamaul to describe "a complete text blindness…although the power of sight, the intellect and the powers of speech are intact.";

1905 – The first U.S. report of childhood reading difficulties is published by Cleveland ophthalmologist Dr. W.E. Bruner.

1963 – Samuel A. Kirk is the first person to use the term "learning disability"; at a conference in Chicago.

1969 – Congress passes the Children with Specific Learning Disabilities Act, which is included in the Education of the Handicapped Act of 1970 (PL 91-230). This is the first time federal law mandates support services for students with learning disabilities.

1975 – The Education for All Handicapped Children Act (PL 94-142), which mandates a free, appropriate public education for all students. (This law is renamed IDEA in 1990.)

1996 – Dr. Guinevere Eden and her research team at the National Institute of Mental Health used functional magnetic resonance imaging (fMRI) – a process that allows us to look at the activity in living brains – to identify the regions of the brain that behave differently in dyslexics.

History of Dyslexia By: LD On Line

ACKNOWLEDGEMENTS

TO GOD
AND ALL MY SIBLINGS.
I DO NOT KNOW WHERE I WOULD BE
NOW WITHOUT ALL OF YOU.

THANKS.

FROM THE AUTHOR

Dear Readers,

In writing this book I have found out a lot about myself, and at the suggestion of a few good friends have decided to add this note of explanation to help with your understanding of my book.

It seems that the way I speak and the way I write are two different entities which is not surprising to all those people in our wide world who suffer from dyslexia. With this impairment, the eyes and the brain do not work together until they are trained to do so. When a lot of us learn to speak it is through our hearing in which we parrot the person to whom we are listening which helps us to sound intelligent.

With this in mind I have decided to insert 6 pages of the edited/unedited manuscript to show how my brain, eyes and hands work together. On the next few pages you will see the edited first and unedited on opposite side. I hope this may help you, my readers, to understand the results any person with a brain disorder is trying to achieve.

Yours Sincerely,

Randymary d Rosier

Author of, Dyslexia: I Live With It!

Readers these pages are edited/non-edited so you can see how dyslexics function.

PREFACE/Edited Pages	Non-Edited Pages
I am dyslexic and dyslexia is a brain disorder that involves the brain, eyes, and hands in that order in my life. Let me show you what I mean I am a writer and I am collecting a sentence in my brain that has the word ***doing*** in it but by the time I have typed the word at least forty to fifty time out of a hundred the word that I put down with my hands come out as **do**.	I am dyslexic and dyslexia is a brain disorder that involves the brain, eyes, and hands in that order in my life. Let me show you what I mean I am a writer and I am collecting a sentence in my brain that has the word doing in it but by the time I have typed the word at least forty to fifty time out of a hundred the word that I put down with my hands come out as do.
I am a very poor speller and always have a computer dictionary right next to my hands to look up the word that do not come spelling-wise, when I want them recalled from my brain for they are mostly stuck just **waiting** for me to pronounce or try to spell them correctly. This does not mean that I	I am a very poor speller and always have a computer dictionary right next to my hands look up the words that do not come spelling-wise, when I want them recalled from my brain, for they are mostly stuck just wait for me to pronounce or to try to spell them correctly. This does not mean that I

do not know how to spell them it just means that the little doors in my brain/head do not want to open up to let the word pass through to my hands.

Okay, before I go any further let me explain what I mean by little doors. You see I **have** to compartmentalize all the words that I have **learned** correctly since probably the second grade and those compartments are the little doors in my brain. Now this is I hope what everyone of us do to keep from going crazy but I believe that as a dyslexic person it is imperative to do this for I feel that once I have **learned**, done, and achieved any new **ideas,** actions and ability, it is in my head from that time on and all I have to do is call it up through the right door.

do not know how to spell them it just means that the little doors in my brain/head do not want to open up to let the word pass through to my hands.

Okay, before I go any further let me explain what I mean by little doors. You see I <u>had</u> to compartmentalize all the words that I have <u>leaned</u> correctly since probably the second grade and those compartments are the little doors in my brain. Now this is I hope what everyone of us do to keep from going crazy but I believe that as a dyslexic person it is imperative to do this for I feel that once I have <u>learn</u>, and achieved any new <u>idea</u>, actions and ability, it is in my head from that time on and all I have to do is call it up through the right door.

Sometimes it never comes and **sometimes** it is very slow in coming and I have to search for another similar word to fill in the gap. But that does not mean that I do not have it memorized somewhere in the gray matter in my brain.

So now let me get back to the brain and hands difficulty. Earlier I used the word *doing* when I was trying to describe the movement from the brain to the hands and that it would have come out as **do**. That is the dyslexia for I do not put endings on the majority of all my **words**. No **ing's**, no **ed's**, or **ly's** and en's my brain just does not react that way.

Does it make a difference in my intelligence? No. But does it make a difference in the mines of let's say a teacher, perspective boss, when writing a book, taking a spelling test or writing a paper for a PhD? Yes. I had to go to a psychologist to get a written document that **stated** that I was dyslexic to get help in the learning center of the university that I attended. So, the professors would not mark me down for **misspellings** on all my class papers or they would not mark up all my paper with **RED** pencil circling the wrong words time after time without my diagnoses. Can you even imagine how frustrating that can be to an adult let alone a child that is trying so hard to get a good grade and it is not even their fault but a malfunction of the brain? What makes it worst is that often people in charge of not give a **damn**.

Now I can almost see some of your brains wanting to state "Well we all have something that is wrong with us."

when writing a book, taking a spelling test or writing a paper for a PhD? Yes. I had to go to a psychologist to get a written document that <u>stated</u> that I was dyslexic to get help in the learning center of the university that I attended. So, the professors would not mark me down for <u>misspelling</u> on all my class papers or they would not mark up all my paper with <u>RED</u> pencil circling the wrong words time after time without my diagnoses. Can you even imagine how frustrating that can be to an adult let alone a child that is trying so hard to get a good grade and it is not even their fault but a malfunction of the brain? What makes it worst is that often people in charge do not give a <u>**dam**</u>.

Now I can almost see some of your brains wanting to state "Well we all have something that is wrong with us."

I would not fault you for thinking it or stating it but that is not going to help the third grader who **wants** to pass his advancement test to the fourth grade but not fully comprehension their third-grade reader yet. We as a society do not leave anyone behind, we pass everyone on to the next grade. I remember a teacher in whose classroom I was helping as a tutor. She had a student that was smart. You could see it in his face the way it **lit** up when he knew that he had gotten the word right when reading out loud.

This youngster had missed kindergarten and half of his first-grade classes due to, (I believe, being new to our country and was placed in the second grade for his age. Also, there was a younger brother in the first-grade.)

He could not spell, he could not read very well, even though he was trying ten-time harder **than** the other students in his efforts, and he was going to be passed to the next grade. His brave teacher endangered her job **by** saying she was not going to sign any document stating he was ready to be passed on, for he was not ready. This is wrong and with just holding him back and taking the second grade over again he would **have** most likely gotten the help that he needed.

It is wrong to advance students to the next grade if they are not ready. But this practice is happening in schools all over the United States and has got to stop.

He could not spell, he could not read very well, even though he was trying ten-time harder <u>then</u> the other students in his efforts, and he was going to be passed to the next grade. His brave teacher endangered her job <u>be</u> saying she was not going to sign any document stating he was ready to be passed on, for he was not ready. This is wrong and with just holding him back and taking the second grade over again he would <u>had</u> most likely gotten the help that he needed.

It is wrong to advance students to the next grade if they are not ready. But this practice is happening in schools all over the United States and has got to stop.

INTRODUCTION

DYSLEXIA: THE EXPERTS DESCRIBE WHAT IT IS

From Socrates forward, teachers have been teaching in the oral style standing at the front of the room before a class of students and speaking to them. Also, since that time, teachers have been teaching to students who are the fastest learners. This appears to have been a set way to teach—always to the fastest learners figuring the rest would catch up. Then in the 1970s there was a great explosion of ideas about how the human brain grows, works, and learns. So, with these medical and physiological advances in understanding the brain, all this data has moved into the training of teachers and psychologists.

Children have a gradual process of brain maturation. Many children's brains reach a certain maturity between the first and third grades. On the other hand, many children's brains do not mature as quickly and about twenty percent seem to be in this group with slower brain maturation. The human brain does not stop growing until the child is twenty years old.

The maturation of a child's brain has nothing to do with intelligence but rather how the human eye perceives or processes information. For example, a child with dyslexia will see letters that transpose their position or move on the page. The child has no control over this perception of the eye. They need only to wait for the brain to mature to correctly align its eyes' perception.

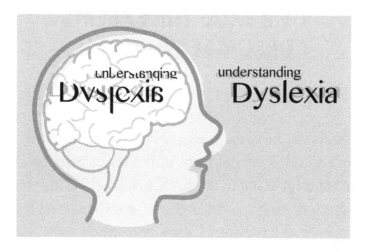

This takes time. However, in the classroom, time is often limited. Students who did not grasp the information as the teacher taught it were often lost, at least for a while. Children without dyslexia do not have this eye perception problem and children with dyslexia are thwarted in their ability to learn as quickly for what the eye tells the brain it sees. Dyslexia does not have anything to do with a child's intelligence. The eye sends information to the brain that may become scrambled because of the brain's lack of maturity. As teachers understood so little about how the brain grows any child who did not learn the way "fast learner" absorbed information became labeled a "slow learner."

"Not only is this not true of children who have dyslexia and other visual perception difficulties, such labeling affects the child's view of themselves, affects the teachers who will teach the child in the next grade, and affects other people's view of the child. For dyslexics understand that they do not get certain information as some of their classmates do, the dyslexic child works harder and harder to grasp what he is missing, (about six times harder than the child who does not have dyslexia!); the child knows she's intelligent but does not know why she is not getting it. The child does not know that the teacher's teaching style is causing her further difficulty regarding her absorption of knowledge. The harder the child tries to learn ways around the learning difficulty, the more tenacity, determination, perseverance and other good characteristics spur the child to keep on working; but it also discourages the child to be perceived as not bright. The child's lack of interest in school heightens for she can never win, despite that the child is working much harder than the child without dyslexia.

Concepts of different teaching styles were developed in the 1970s and teachers who were educated during these years learned to teach the child according to the child's best way of learning. Now teachers know that how they teach affects how the child learns and try to adjust their style to the best way a child can learn from them.

Because we didn't know how the brain worked we could not teach differently in the generation we grew up in, but since the explosion of learning in the 70s, college students educated to be teachers now know better in the 90s and better teaching is being done. The child just needs individual help in certain areas to learn what she missed because of dyslexia. So, if the child is taken from the mainstream class and allowed to catch up in the area of phonics, though, let us say, one half hour a day of phonics…then the child can learn what she missed and move on with her classmates…. And the specialist can work with her on third-grade materials that are relevant to what her classmates are learning. It is an unfilled gap in knowledge that needs to be filled which will allow the child to move forward with her grade. They simply need to be re-taught particular concepts." *Learning Specialist Eve Bass' discussion on Dyslexia, 8/30/07, while working in the Peace Corps, Manila, Philippines.*

It is important to note that in many cases a child who has dyslexia never grows out of that condition but learns different "tricks" to help them cope.

Many researchers believe that children diagnosed with dyslexia after the third grade will always need to be aware of their own learning style. That is one of the positive outcomes of research findings in the area of brain function that gives these children skills that better enable them to succeed.

In the area of creativity there are many dyslexics in history who show giftedness in the area of creativity. Einstein was one, but the list is long.

Bill Gates, a well-known dyslexic, stated, "Dyslexia causes difficulties in learning to read, write and spell. Short-term memory, mathematics, concentration, personal organization and sequencing may also be affected, usually arising from a weakness in the processing of language-based information. Biological in origin, it tends to run in families, but environmental factors also contribute. It can occur at any level of intellectual ability. It is not the result of poor motivation, emotional disturbance, sensory impairment or lack of opportunities, but it may occur alongside any of these. The effect of dyslexia can be largely overcome by skilled, specialist teaching and the use of compensatory strategies."

Bill Gates, speaking at the Dyslexia Institute, November 2, 2002. Reported by: JAMAICAOBSERVER.COM

CHAPTER ONE

BRAIN MALFUNCTION NAMED

Okay, to start out this book I am going to try to give you my story in chronological order the best I can remember. Growing up in the family, schooling, then into the business world and ending with writing this book.

It is really strange to live with the unknown and still know that there is something not right with you. I knew that I was intelligent and came from two families where there were no slouches in the brain areas of life. I have strong genes from many generations of doctors, lawyers, inventors, teachers, plumbers, writers, farmers, adventurers, and women who were strong great leaders and I wondered why I was not living up to the genes that must also be flowing through my veins. It always felt like my life was one step forward and two steps back. I do all right in the arts but you cannot make it in this life without math and reading. I rarely got a grade higher than an "S" for satisfactory or a "C+." Even with a higher education and rising to the level of a senior administrator before quitting the business world that feeling that I should be doing better never left my mind and ego until the day many years later that I learned the answer.

That special day came when my sister who had had a similar situation to mine growing up (but to her advantage she learned how to read people, especially teachers) was describing learning difficulties one of their children was having in school. Knowing that help was needed, she initiated testing and then was asked to take some tests herself. After the results of the testing was completed my sister visiting our mother was relating what help was need to help bring the grades up to par. I happened to arrive home from work at the time they were talking and sat down to listen. After all the gleaned information was explained, I heard for the first time the word "dyslexic." But before I could even ask my first question, my sister turned to me and said, "And Randy you are dyslexic, too."

Here I was forty-two years old and for the first time in my life I knew what was wrong with me. I was DYSLEXIC! Wow, did my life start to change after that, for I had my education behind me and had started to use the strengths that I had built up in myself for the first time. Even my mother said that finding out that my life's disorder had a name changed my outlook.

I will never be rid of dyslexia. I will always be unable to do higher math, I will always have to read a paragraph in a book several times to get the full meaning, and most likely will have to look up the meaning of thousands of words. I will never be able to write a paper or book without having someone else edit it for me. But, I have learned that my brain and eye see two different forms when relating to each other and this knowledge has empowered me.

CHAPTER TWO

FAMILY

I grew up just like any other middle-class child. There were my four siblings to play with and the minds of five was always more fertile for fun. When we wanted more activity, there were more than twenty kids within our radius of home with always some activity until the light was fading and the moms were calling us in for the night.

Summers meant playing games like Kick the Can, Red Rover, and Hide and Seek in the street. Being raised at the end of the Second World War within a neighborhood of lots of kids our age was not only convenient but also safe.

I remember one night after dinner when the five of us were playing with the kids of the block and having a great time. Then mom called for us to come in and one of us called back, "Oh just ten more minutes, Mom, it's not even dark out yet." We got our ten minutes and then everyone went inside for the night. My mother was the gauge ruler for the block and most of the parents went by what she let us do.

When I was between twelve and thirteen my mom's mother moved in to live with us. I have often thought about those years. Having grams within the house's group until the week before she died was both a pleasure and a threat.

She was a disciplinarian, not like my mother at all, who was a lot easier to understand. Mom was Gram's oldest child and was already widowed, when Gram moved in. Putting together the two different personalities of two strong women under one roof made for a very interesting life.

Grandma had only an eighth-grade education and had had a very successful working career and in demand where she went before she married a doctor. She was what I would call "street smart" for she educated herself with every means she had at her disposal. Though I never heard my Grams sing I was told that she had a wonderful voice. She had received a learning scholarship to Vienna as a young woman but being raised in the time of the great depression all hands were need at home to care for the family.

The only reason I mention this is because I still wonder how I would have learned my multiplication and division tables with my poor brain for math if it had not been for Gram. Now, I can remember all of the grammar and math drillings all of us got over and over again until we learned whatever we needed.

Wonderful for me for her instincts must have sensed the help I needed. I do remember that it took a long time for me to get the multiplication tables down, and sometimes I still have to go back to the fives or tens tables and count forward if I get stuck.

It is very eerie but I can see my grams standing by the sink in the kitchen peeling potatoes and hear her saying "6x7=, 9x8=," as I try to learn them. There was also the time that she would ask me to spell **animal** or **Jupitar** and would split the syllable's up so I could hear them also. The one I remember the best was the word (**CHOC O LATE**) chocolate.

※ ※ ※

As the second oldest of the five, with an older brother, I remember around the age of eight I started letting my sister, two and half year's younger, take over my responsibilities for my age while I settled into a very nice dream-like stage where I just stepped back and let things happen. For example, as my sisters and I got older, our mom taught us how to take care of the house when she was at work, including cooking and cleaning. Now I'm not saying I did not do my jobs that were required. It was just that I let my sister do more. This sister is a type A personality, and I found it easy to let her take over. I must say in my defense that when it first started I was not aware that I was doing it but I am sure she just stepped up to the position. I let her become the oldest sister.

Eventually I began to feel that things were starting to move too fast and I was not sure I could keep up. I believe that I felt that something was wrong with me. I did not join in with the rest of the kids in the neighborhood as much as my siblings did. I did not mind being by myself a lot of the time. I was introverted and quiet. At an early age, I retired into my own world for shelter and relief and let the rest of the world circle around me only interacting when it was necessary.

This also was the time, when I was eight, that my father got sick and then he died at the age of thirty-seven and it was traumatic. But I do member a wonderful incident a year earlier that I would like to relate to you to give you a little insight into that loving man my father. I was seven I believe and had to have my tonsils out and was in the hospital most of one day having it done. After work dad came to pick my mother and me up to take us home. I do not remember the ride home but when we got there, dad picked me up and carried me inside. My father was 6 feet plus and I took after him being tall for my age and all legs. He maneuvered us up the stairs to my bedroom and placed me gently on the bed.

Even though I knew the implications of death and was sad, I also had a very strong mother to care for me. I do not think I felt the sense of loss, after his death, then as much as I do now especially after writing this book.

Where I fit into this scheme of life and what would have happened to me if I did not have the family I grew up in I really do not want to think too long about. All through those early years of my growing up I felt that I was being protected and helped too much even if my family did not know that they were doing it.

My siblings growing up were the best friends anyone could have. Sure, we fought but by the time we went to bed it was all forgotten. I remember one time when the local theater had a Walt Disney movie and Mom said that my sisters and I could go. It must have been in the summer on a Saturday for this was never allowed during the school week and then not very often for Mom could not afford it. The long and short of the story is that unknown to us the theater was showing three movies that day for the price of one. Mom gave me forty cents so we could get in to the movie at five cents and have a nickel treat. We sat through all three movies and had a wonderful time. But Mom was just frantic and had called the theater several times and almost called the police wondering where we were. When we came out of the movies it was dark and we talked and laughed as we walked the three blocks home. What a great day I had without the worries of having always to learn through reading, for I got through that afternoon with my ears, eyes and the love of my sisters' company.

I have always been full of the adventure of life and took risks when I felt it might be fun or interesting. So, between the ages of ten and three my younger sisters and I decided to make a fort in the attic. First, let me describe the house I grew up in.

We lived in a three-story colonial house. It was all white, with four pillars across the front, a blue-shingled roof and plenty of grass all around. We had lived in this house since I was five and I loved the big rooms with their high ceilings. The best place in the whole house to build our fort was in the slightly dark attic. There was one bedroom in the attic and the rest of the floor space outside the room was wide open and dusty. Above the bedroom ceiling was a space and then the sloping eaves. In this space, my sisters and I set up our fort and reached it by the bunk bed ladder. The only bad part of the fort was that the ladder did not reach all the way up the wall, so we had to reach up and then pull ourselves up to the space. It probably would have terrified our mother if she knew.

I went up last and came down first, for someone had to hold the ladder so it would not slip. Since I was the tallest and oldest, it was up to me to help the others up and down each time. We never had any accidents and as soon as I got a little older the fort was abandoned and the ladder was put back with the bunk beds.

Here there could have been a big problem for one of the systems in many dyslexics, is the lack of balance. I was lucky that time none of us got hurt. My balance is and never will be the best. I always thought that my brain was a little off to the right for I have always seemed to glide to the right a few steps when walking down the street and I try to remember to always take the right side when walking with anyone. I never hurt myself but can get black and blue quite a lot.

My brother, who is the oldest and I did not do as much together until we were closer to being adults but he was always there for me. He taught me to dance, sometimes even took me to the sock hops at the high school, and tried to teach me how to drive, but that didn't work out too well. (I learned through driving classes.) The thing we do together now that I love is going to see adventure movies, the ones that have you on the edge of your seat and sometimes screaming out loud.

"Everything in the Right Place" www.dyslexia-kids.com Davis

CHAPTER THREE

SCHOOL

My grandfathers were a doctor and a plumber who owned his own business. My grandmother was a Secretary- Stenographer, who was sought after wherever she worked. Dad's mother had nine children, working alongside of her husband to raise smart children who succeeded in their lives. My father was a Lawyer and owned his own advertising business and mother raised five of us and taught for many years after my father's death. In one of the main areas of learning growing up was that education was stressed as very important. I did not know that my mother refused to even consider putting me in special education classes when it was suggested to her that I was in need of help. She knew that children mature at different stages and sensed I needed extra time for brain growth. She did not start me in kindergarten until I was six and I was half a year older than the other kindergartners but I did not find anything too unusual about learning or making friends. I walked six blocks by myself to the blue door of the school for kindergarten and most of those friends I would be with right through the first year of high school.

Yes, school was not the easiest—my favorite time in the early years was hearing stories and found that I remembered most of them as told. But if asked to read a book or just pick one out to read it was a difficult task. I hoped the teacher never asked me to read out loud for the big words never came very easily to me and I would get stumped on them. Then, after a few minutes, the teacher would move on to someone else which relieved me so I could go back to listening and comprehending. Spelling, reading, and math were my downfall from the fourth grade on and, to some degree, are still troublesome.

Until the age of eight I do not remember much unhappiness or difference in my life. School was good. Fourth grade brought on trouble with the lack of reading well, spelling and the confidence in myself that I knew more vocabulary than how to spell words than I was giving myself credit for. The dyslexia started to show up in my work more and more from then on. I fell into the habit of doing what I could to get along. I now realized that my fourth-grade teacher took me for being slower so she passed me by on a lot of reading. I know now that if I had been able to understand my teachers and what they wanted from me, life would have been a great deal easier to deal with.

Growing up I do not remember my mother ever hassling me about my grades most of which were in the average range except for math, spelling, and reading which were never too good. But not all was bad because after choosing to sit in the first-row close to the blackboard it was suggested that I might need glasses. So, at about the age of eight I got a pair of pink-framed glasses that I thought made my eyes, my best feature, look even bigger.

Then, at the age of twelve my eye sight improved and I threw them in a drawer and did not wear glasses again until I was in my fifties. But I sure liked those glasses.

Another thought just slipped in to mind about pain or loneliness that followed me through grade school was when I heard my classmates talking about me and calling me names. I pretended not to hear or just stuffed it away, saying to myself that it did not matter anyway. But it did matter and I know now that what they were saying was abusive and bullying even though they never thought of it that way. For it was just a way to describe me, but it did hurt. With my denial and submerging of my pain I did not recognize how much it hurt or how much effect it had on me until I started writing this book. The pointing fingers, the giggling after I made a mistake, the toleration of me in the group but never fully accepted. The girls who were trying to make points with their group by pointing out something I did wrong. Yes, I was probably too sensitive and did not always speak up for myself but that was not the easiest thing to do when your self-esteem is non-existent.

One of the hateful incidents that happened during the summer in the sixth or seventh grade at summer camp is hard to forget. I had not brought enough pads for my menstrual cycle and ran out, staining my underpants.

One of the popular females of the group, or so she thought, announced out aloud that I had my period and did not even know it. I responded that I did know, thank you very much, but ran out of pads. Unfortunately for me I did not think of going to the nurse and asking for help.

It was hurtful to realize that everyone in my class knew who the smart kids were and the ones who always had trouble learning. Because of this, it seemed I was always on the edge of two different groups. I was partially accepted by the smart girls (the boys never seemed too important until seventh and eighth grade) but I was placed in the lower group that learned differently. This puzzled me for I knew that I was smart but I was never able to get better grades in most subjects and Mother would just tell me to do my best. To this day I am so glad that she did not pin that label of Special Ed. Even though it might have done me good on the learning side it would never have been good for my self-esteem, which was and still is not the best and even now often brings pain when least expecting it.

CHAPTER FOUR

"YOU ARE NOT COLLEGE MATERIAL"

I was an intelligent kid and dyslexia has nothing to do with I.Q. but with brain and eye coordination. The eye sees a word on a page and sends it to the brain. The brain takes it in and sees it totally different due to the lack of maturity and sends it back as completely different, scrambled. So, the learner has to learn each word by rote. You have to remember that there was not a lot known about dyslexia in the U.S. until the late forties and fifties. My learning was taking an object like a pencil and recognizing it then given the word spell out, **PENCIL**, was the way I learned to read.

I am sure there are people out there that are dyslexic and were called all the unkind names that the slower students were called while in school. I was called all the names too, but I must have just let them ride over me or stuffed them into the back of my memory. This only isolated me more from making a lot of real close friends, and I cannot remember life's importance outside of school other than being with my family.

I probably knew how to read pretty well for the first grade but I did not read much. In our home, there were always books to page through or read and I loved nursery rhymes, which I can recite by heart to this day. I think that books that I pick up for fun stopped in the fourth grade. The stronger feeling that I was not reading up to my peers and not getting the grades that I thought I should put pressure on me to read nothing but the textbooks that I had too. I was not really treated differently by my peers but I do remember the fourth-grade teacher and I did not get along. Not that she was mean to me, but maybe she sensed something was wrong and did not know how to help so she just let me be. I was working at my age capacity and achieving but bored, for the lessons did not interest me so I think I tuned off and it was never caught. By the time I turned back on it was too late. As a result, I have had a struggle all my life in education and jobs.

By eighth grade, my teacher was not content to let me be. This particular teacher, even though I cannot remember her name, and have forgiven her many times over the years humiliated me. I still remember the incident as if it was yesterday. I was standing at the blackboard trying to do a math problem and having a hard time. While most of the class was starting on beginning Algebra, I was still counting on my fingers to get hopefully the right answer to complete my task. The teacher joined me at the board and then, after looking over my work, said loud enough for everyone to hear, "Do not think about going to college, you're not college material."

I am sure I was talked to that way many times over the years by many teachers, but this is the only one my brain held on to. I have a university degree and maybe that teacher unconsciously planted the will for me to get my degree that very day. Even though it took a long time to achieve, I never gave up.

A dyslexic can have trouble learning in many areas and mine were mostly in reading and math. I just had enough energy to get through my classes and get grades at a passing level to graduate. My high school years at St. Paul Central are a blur. Again, due to the reading and understanding the text that was required for passing. This did not leave too much time to join many extra-curricular activities and get to know new people because I was never asked to any of the dances or out for a date from my peer at school.

College was never one of the areas that I tried too hard to fight for and it was not because I did not think I could make it. It just did not interest me.

So, I decided to help my country and joined the newly started group called VISTA (Volunteer In Service To America). After three months of training in Syracuse, New York in the Head Start, part of the government's program, I was told that there were no more spaces and asked to go home.

"They said they would call me when a space opened up."

"I said, If I go home I will not be back, so put me in another program."

At the time, the only space left for a volunteer was at St. Mary's Colin Anderson Center in West Virginia, the Mental Retardation Area, now called, *Special Needs*. If I did not fit right in there, I do not think I would have fit anywhere.

The hardest part about being around the employees of Colin Anderson was to learn how to deal with the fears we volunteers seemingly brought with us. The staff feared that the three of us assigned to help them were there to take over their jobs and that really hit home on my rethinking that I really needed college for my own future.

By this time, several years after high school, I was fitting into society as well as any high school degree-holding student could and that September, after returning home, at the age of twenty-two I was enrolled as a freshman in college.

That did give me an advantage though, for I had a working/volunteer back ground that most students right out of high school did not have. But I knew from experience learning was not going to come easy as for each eighteen- or nineteen-year-olds. I would have to work six times harder to get what came much easier to them and not because of being out of practice but because of the dyslexia.

Unfortunately, college at that time was not to be very long lived, for after two years I was losing ground fast with poor grades and sleep walking.

After seeing a doctor about my sleeping problem, it was suggested that I get out of school before I hurt myself in my sleep, which the doctors attributed to stress. But I did promise myself that if I ever found a college or university that would let me choose the classes that I wanted to take I would go back. I was going to prove that eighth grade teacher wrong.

Metropolitan State University here I come.

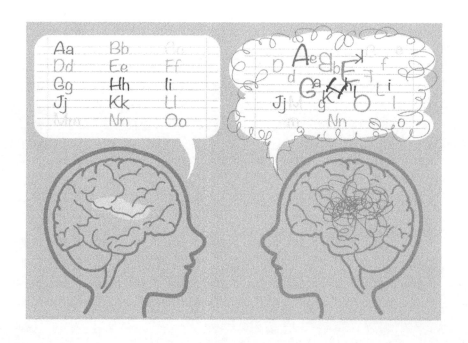

CHAPTER FIVE

VENTURING OUT

The age of twenty-six brought big changes in my life. I started having success with my life outside of work and family. But first I would like to tell you what started this change. You see I had a great aunt who was probably a success in her life but did not seem that way to me. She was a school teacher in kindergarten, had never married, and kept house for her brother and father for many years. I really got to know her after she was retired and moved in to live with my family.

She had been living in a one-room boarding house after being shoved around from relative to relative upon the death of her father. The boarding house got too expensive which brought her moving in with us. She joined my mother, my grandmother, who was her sister-in-law, my three sisters and me. We had a small room at the top of the stairs that became my aunt's room that she seldom left except for meals. This way of life was the habit that she was quite used to when she was in the boarding house so it was nothing new to her. But it had an effect on me. I do believe that my aunt was very introverted only shined when she was with children for she was always happy around my sisters and I when we were younger.

Staying in that little room most of the day doing nothing would have driven me mad, but it did not seem to affect her at all. After seeing this for some time, I decided that I had to do something with my life. I was already introverted enough and realized what could happen to me if I did not do something fast.

First, it was time to get my driver's license. I lived three blocks south of home on one bus line and four blocks north on another. Driving was not really necessary to get around but the knowledge would help my ego immensely. Next, I have always loved to swim and decided to take a scuba diving class at the YMCA. It turned out that I was the only female with seven males and that was a very interesting class. Yes, I am a certified scuba diver but don't do much diving now. Then started traveling by myself once every year, and this started changing my life.

Traveling alone is not the most fun, but after viewing my great aunt's way of life and knowing that I did not want to live that way speared me on. My first trip let me know that I did have the strength to do what I had to do to get me through planning a trip, getting to my destination, through the trip itself, and back home. With each trip, I gained the strength that had been lost through years of fighting with my dyslexia and chopping away at my self-esteem.

First, at the age of nineteen, I lived and went to school in Mexico City for six months. Even though I was still not fully on my own for I lived with my father's sister and that was a great help I saw how other people live, learned to get around Mexico City, gained self-esteem and retained two subjects: chess and beginner's Spanish. To this day I can still speak enough broken Spanish to be understood and play chess with some wins.

Remembering, that by gaining the ups and downs, wins and defeats, of my unchallenged brain for so many years, I knew I needed to change from introverted to extroverted if I was going to succeed.

What inspired the learning of the game of chess? After thinking about it I have come to the knowledge that it is the strategy, the thinking of the correct moves and how can I out fox my opponent and win? Winning is not all important but it sure helped when the feelings of defeat most of the time creeps in. Winning gave me a boost that challenged me on to keep fighting against anything that held me back and helped me gain a strong feeling for adventure that I have never lost.

On a trip to Guatemala the plane was hit by lighting and forced to land for several hours for safety reasons which made my next connection and arrival three hours late. There was no group of nine women who were going to be my traveling companions for the next two weeks waiting for me. I then realized upon arrival that my itinerary was still on my bed in Minnesota. What to do when the sky was already turning dark and I did know the name of my hotel?

Help came in the form of the man sitting next to me on the flight down to Guatemala, a very nice man living in the U.S., visiting home. He had lost his luggage. Fate stepped in and on spying him I went over and I explained my plight. He introduced me to his sister and mother, neither of whom spoke a lot of English, but with his sister's Spanish and my English and a local phone we got my itinerary and me to my hotel.

Then being informed there was no group in the hotel under the names I had and no rooms, so I was alone again. I found out after some questioning with my broken Spanish that there was a room for one hundred dollars for the night. I took it: The next morning I missed my first flight into the interior and got there five hours later, which meant that again I missed my tour group. After arriving late, I had to switch on my Spanish, make another collect call for the next stopping place, but finally arrived at my destination.

The most surprising part about the entire adventure was telling my new travel companions my tale and finding out that they all agreed in the same circumstances, they would have caught the next plane back to the U.S. I struck another blow against dyslexia for staying with it and not missing a great adventure.

Traveling was what changed me the most, for it not only saved my sanity but was how I found self-strength outside of my family.

CHAPTER SIX

COPING

Have you ever been writing a letter or a paper for a class and you get a great word that will just finish the sentence? It happens to me all the time, and if I do not know how the word is spelt and for the life of me cannot find the word in the dictionary from the many different ways that I try spelling it, I give up in frustration and write a less descriptive word. Now multiply that by ten and you get the feeling I often have when I sit down to write. That is why the dictionary is always at my fingertips. Oh yeah, I hear you all saying, why not use Spell Check, and the answer is that too many words in the English language can have similar meanings but different spellings. If I want the word **their** in a sentence: "This was Sue and Tom's first car and was **there** pride and joy," you know that the word you wanted was their but Spell Check does not substitute their, for, there, for it is spelt correctly and so does not show up as wrong. This example is an easy reversal, but what about the words spgettie/spaghetti, oveous/obvious, and the word devastated. I spell words correctly when I pronounce them correctly, but some words are a constant frustration for I cannot find them in the dictionary the way I pronounce them.

Often, by the time I figure that out—for I am not always on the computer—I lose my sense of what I was trying to write.

When it comes to my method of learning it was quite different then it is today. First, I had to learn everything by rote and then when the schools started to use <u>phonetics</u> which are the tools for spelling. I have to admit that I only remember one year in grade school that they were taught and I did not catch on to the concept. Now in my later years I have learned to break down the sound of speech and am able to pronounce the word correctly. With this concept learned, I am able to spell the words or find it in the dictionary.

Then there was also, <u>Letter reversals</u> which is still a problem. Especially with the letter T and R, d and b, the vowels e and a. Such as the words: <u>then</u> or <u>than</u>, <u>bed</u> and <u>bad</u> and <u>out</u> and <u>our.</u>

Nevertheless, there are some good things that come out of having dyslexia. Once a recollection of any item is placed into the brain it is in there for good. It may take a few minutes to recall all you know about the subject—I call this the doors in my brain that have to be opened and searched through to find what I'm looking for—but eventually you find it. Let me give you an example: Driving directions. I am very poor at figuring out which way I have to go, especially when driving, so I have to get exact information. If someone starts telling me how to get to a certain building, town, or mall, I have to write it down or have them write it out. Then I must be sure that they say turn left or right on to a specific street and not east or south, for what is east when driving in many different directions? But the good thing is, once I have driven someplace I can always find it again without difficulty or even tell someone else how to get there. You may say that everyone has this difficulty once in a while, and I know that they do, but does panic kick in every time the information is not exact and you have to go miles out of your way before you can find the next place to get help?

Here is a little story. As I've said, I am a person filled with the love of adventure. One of my nephew's daughters was getting married in another state that I had never visited, a place where you just did not hail a cab once you got out of the airport. No, I had many, many miles to go, so I rented a car and started out. I did have directions but there was a turn-about that had to be maneuvered. I was at least ten miles down the freeways of Montana before I started thinking that I had messed up on the turn-about. So what do you do when home and business are far between each other in this state and there is no cell phone? You start searching for a house or business and I found one house and drove in to ask directions, and thank goodness, I did for the people where just delightful. The wife realized right away what I had done and said she would take me back to the turn-about and get me in the right direction. Then she said, "My husband and I go to that town you want quite often and since you have come this far, why not just keep going and I will write down the exact directions and towns that you have to go through to get to where you want to go." It worked, but that is not the way to start a vacation.

There are many other good things that dyslexics might say is good about this brain disorder. I think you learn to take life in a calmer manner. Sure, I get frustrated when something that is planned does not go off the way it should and I get lost, or get a flat tire, or even get a drink dumped on a brand-new dress, which, though surprising, I just take in stride and think, oh it's washable so do not worry, and go on enjoying myself.

To the dyslexic these happenings can be big, but each time something happens to me, at least I found that it became a little easier to accept and start again with the memories intact so it would be a lot easier the second time. Yes, there were many times that I repeated the same mistakes—people's names take three times to get stuck in my brain waves—but how many of you can say that after the third time of hearing a name you can remember that person's name forever?

Over the last twenty years, ever since I learned what the disorder was called, I have talked to anyone who asked, what is dyslexia? Now I have not done this in a formal setting, but I have read and collected articles I could find on what the experts had to say about the subject. I have found that even though there are doctors, physiologists, and authors who have written on the subject of dyslexia, not too many actually have dyslexia, while I, on the other hand, live with it.

Even though you live day in and day out with not being able to fully use your perceived intelligence, you learn to live with the one that God gave you. After all, for me it was handed down through generations of de Rosier brains. No one even knew why some of my family members had a brain that did not function correctly for generations, or why, in the early nineteen-forties, this problem was not being investigated by the learned people of the medical fields. People who exhibited dyslexic symptoms were just labeled slow.

I heard many times since I was a teenager from different members of the de Rosier family. I cannot exactly tell you what I did to make someone tell me as a warning not to do things that would disgrace me in public. I was never alert enough to ask what I did to receive this warning, but the admonition that I heard was close to this: "Oh do not act that way or someone might take you as a slow de Rosier."

For many years I wondered what a, "Slow de Rosier was" but it was not until I was in my forties that I finally figured out the meaning. The slow de Rosier were the people who throughout the generations did not get help, did not get educated, who were probably kept at home, never to marry, probably laughed at and shut away. Why? For they had the brain disorder called dyslexia. Without help, they never went to school, never read, maybe never even went to church, and most likely led a very solitary life. But at least I hope they were loved.

CHAPTER SEVEN

UNIVERSITY

Though it took ten years of night school, I got my degree.

I returned to schooling in my fifties at Metropolitan State University. I barely had finished two years in my twenties when I quit for medical reasons but life had showed me that getting my degree would be another lift to my self-esteem and working power.

I decided not to go back into Education but took the university's General College classes instead. These were classes that I chose in the GC theme. It was pretty clear sailing especially with curriculum courses like English, Algebra, and Spanish finished. Taking classes like <u>Music in the Twin Cities</u> where we attended concerts and operas then wrote about our experience in what we heard, how it influences our opinion of good or bad music.

Another class that I really enjoyed was <u>Photography</u>, one of my favorite photo under the title of "Black on White"; with a scene of the back second floor porch of our house in the shadows of the sun and shade coming through the porch door that lead off my bedroom. The photo was taken from the inside and many plants from inside and out are seen. It was all dark inside and a wonderful sunny day out which showed up my class work to the point that I got an "A" on the photo. Now this may not relate to my dyslexia except that my ego and self-esteem went soring.

I had it framed.

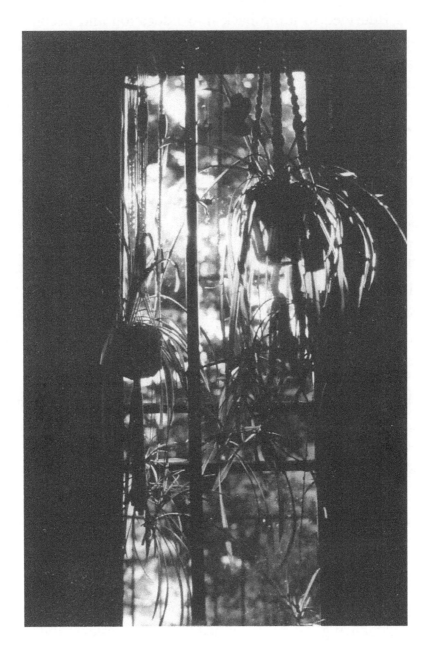

Study in Black and White Photography Class 2007

Then the university decided to add Education to their format and I decided to jump back into Education and become a teacher and almost starting all over again in getting my degree. This is also when the real problems with my dyslexia started showing its ugly head again.

Being dyslexic often brings with it the inability to spell. The misspelling of words is not really the dyslexics fault for the brain in many cases has not learned the difference. This must be very frustrating for a person who is reading my work so I would let the teachers know that I was dyslexic.

The hardest unfairness for me before confirmation of my disability was when I wrote a paper, had someone check it over, and still got a lower grade for misspellings. Some of my professors did not count down for misspellings, but I would get notes, "Why don't you check out the learning center?"

The learning center had to have proof that you have a disability to help you. In my junior year at Metropolitan State I finally did go to see a psychologist and took all the tests to confirm that I really was dyslexic. Why it took me so long I really cannot tell you except that maybe it finally sank into my brain that without documentation I would always get lower grades no matter how hard I worked.

Still, there were times that even with the confirmation of dyslexia I got marked down. I always started each new class, by introducing myself, explained that I was dyslexic and that one of my biggest problems was that I cannot spell. Hoping I would not be marked down, I said, sometimes my papers might have incorrect words on them even though I have them edited before I turn them in.

I had one professor who either had no understanding of dyslexia or just did not care. I was marked down on every paper I handed in to this professor and also the paper looked like it had been through the war of RED pencil. I finally took my documents in and stuck them under the professor's nose and said, "If you do not stop marking my paper up and lowering my grade, I will go to the Dean of the University and have you brought up on charges, for not going along on the requirements for people with disabilities guidelines. I will give you one week to change my grade to show the whole semester of my work as it should be." I got what I needed but never took another class by that professor. I learned the hard way how to fight for myself.

CHAPTER EIGHT

DIAGNOSED TO GET HELP

I not only earned my degree at Metropolitan State University, had an official diagnosis of dyslexia and a description of the disorder as it affected me.

The following excerpts are from the report by my Licensed Psychologist on August 12, 2001. I am including this for the reasons that it might help some readers understand the difficulties that I and other dyslexics have and the need for accommodations to smooth the way in learning.

"REASON FOR REFERRAL:" Ms. Randymary de Rosier a 57-year-old, single, Caucasian female majoring in Education at Metropolitan State University stated she carries a 2.62 grade point average. She works for the St. Paul Public School System. She reported a learning disability, first diagnosed in childhood. Presenting problems include reversal of order of numbers and letters, poor spelling, pronouncing words incorrectly, problems writing word endings and difficulty with math. She reports requiring extra time to complete reading and math assignments. Her goal is to become "a good educational teacher." She was referred for a psychological evaluation in order to assess cognitive functioning, intentional functioning and achievement for the purpose of educational learning center help and time and a half for all testing in a separate quiet room.

Vocational: For many years she worked in the banking system as a teller, receptionist/ secretary at an electric company and ended her business career as an assistant to the president of an insurance company. Finally found her true vocation in the school system.

Problem on the job: This included having to look up the spelling of words in the dictionary, difficulty correctly solving math word problems, confusing the digits 6 and 9, reversing the sequence of digits, slow pace due to needing to check for errors, reversing numbers so often asking if she may repeat the numbers back. She stated that she hated typing for "I hit the wrong keys or bunch letters." It took longer than average to learn new procedures, but retaining all information once she learns it. She stated that she had excellent work quality and got along with all coworkers or supervisors.

TEST INTERPRETATIONS: Ms. Randymary de Rosier is majoring in Education at a Metropolitan State University. She recalls lifelong struggles to master reading, writing and mathematics. She reports compensation for learning difficulties by frequent checking, frequent use of a dictionary, use of a calculator, asking others to reread her work for errors.

Functional Limitations:

Recognizing faces;

Slow pace in the work place due to need to check work frequently;

Borderline deductive reasoning, special relations and non-verbal reasoning;

Borderline visual sequential memory;

Errors in simple mathematical calculations due to confusing similar looking digits, reversing and rotating digits, reversing the order of digits;

Poor motor memory and motor sequential memory resulting in excessive errors typing;

Frequent spelling errors in business and personal writing.

REASONABLE ACCOMMODATIONS TO ALLOW THE STUDENT TO BEST DEMONSTRATE HER KNOWLEDGE.

1. It is recommended that the test format be modified to allow the client to write her answers directly in the test booklet due to visual processing deficits including rotating and reversing letters and numbers and borderline visual sequential memory. Provision of a test scribe to transfer the student's answers to the record form is also recommended.
2. On testing, points should not be deducted for writing, mechanics errors, unless writing mechanics is directly

being tested. She should be permitted to compose on a word processor with spelling and grammar check to answer essay questions.
3. Double extended time should be provided for essay questions due to Word Fluency.
4. In testing mathematics, extended time might result in a mild improvement in her test scores for she has an inability to master mathematic concepts, such as how to multiply fractions. Permission to refer to a list of mathematical formula is recommended.

Ten years—that was how long it took me to get my degree and a lot of that time was at night school. I was working full time when I made the decision to take the diploma and get out of the classroom. But throughout all those years I had a lot of trouble in the business world with the functional limitations diagnosed by the psychologist, with what I had to fight against in every job. Take a look at some of the jobs I held over the years:

A company that helped citizens with disabilities

Chiropractic office

Credit union

3 banks

5 temporary services

2 insurance companies

2 real estate companies

3 department stores

Store detective

2 universities as receptionists

Bottling company

2 companies that make rubber stamps and tool.

Law Office

Administrative Assistant for insurance company

Para Educator within the Public-School System

All these positions from teller to administrative assistant made up my business world and I never made much over thirty thousand. But the stress of holding on to those jobs as long as I could is what I am trying to show here. The longest position I held, except for the last, was for five years. Please do not misunderstand me, for I was happy in most of the positions that I held and learned a lot getting confidence and knowledge with each new situation.

The jewel of the positions I held was working for the St. Paul School System. Even though I never was licensed as a teacher for the lack of not passing the Minnesota license test in Math, missing it by four points after taking it six time. But in the position that I acquired there I understood the students I worked with, who had learning challenges for I was one of them. You see I was in my element for I felt I had finally found the position that I was longing for.

On the other hand, I also volunteered most of my life—it was one of the expected avenues that the family just did and it was also one of the areas that I excelled in and enjoyed. The first one I remember is work with the Red Cross and handed out bulletins to get people in giving blood, I was not able to give my own blood for I was anemic so this was the next best way to help.

Volunteering, why this? Because this was the area that I most felt comfortable using my talents, where I would be helping out and getting some real success without having the feeling of that hard struggle that I had to keep up. The adults and children that I helped were eager to learn and as they grew in their confidence so did I.

The one success that was the most memorable and that I will never forget was helping a third grader whose parents came from Somalia and even though he was born here I expect the language spoken at home was not English. He was struggling with reading and the meaning of words. We had one hour twice a week outside of the classroom to get his word meaning and reading stronger. He remembered and understood what I was teaching him very quickly and with flash cards and books for his mental age he improved very fast even to his teacher surprise.

I was using flash cards with him during one lesson and he was getting them all right. Now on the cards were pictures of items like a hat and he was supposed to spell the word. Not realizing the paper was thin and he could see the spelling on the other side.

After going through about six cards he started to laugh and I asked why and he said, "I can see the spelling through the card.

Then there was one day that I came for his session and he was out of sorts and even though he left with me he would not participate. Lucky, I had a new book on machines, that he really enjoyed knowing about, so I just started reading the story and before long he grabbed the book and read for the rest of the hour.

When it came time for me to move on he said, "You cannot leave you are my best teacher." One more win for my side.

CHAPTER NINE

FINDING MY VOICE

Dyslexia has not been an easy disorder to live with. Even now, as an adult who has somewhat recovered, *for a dyslexic will never fully recover,* into a life that has been successful and meaningful, there is still the pain that keeps drifting back.

My understanding about this mental disability is that by the third grade if a child has not been tested by a license physiologist when the parents or guardians think there is a possibility of dyslexia, that it should be done quickly and every eight years after while in school. When I started in school, the existence of this brain disorder was barely heard of and so most students that could not function or process the written word were considered slow or handicapped and put in special classes. After this, the child was labeled "Special Education" and treated that way all through their school life.

Thanks to a progressive mother who realized that children developed differently and at their own pace and refused to put me in a special education class. After working in special education for ten years, some thirty plus years later I am half and half on her decision, for special education may have helped me learn faster. I do know that I suffered the entire gambit of wrong information for the lack of knowledge and help.

Yes, with the feelings of pain that I feel even now as I look back to write this book. Because I knew that I was smart but just could not get the good grades or get rid of the feeling that there was something wrong.

* * *

All my life my rhythms have been much slower. I did not get my driver's license until I was twenty-six, but we were living between two bus stops which made it easier to get to my destinations. I also had several siblings that drove cars before I got my license and would take me anywhere I needed to be. This continuation of the protection or enabling as I see it now was a mistake but I did not know how to stop it. This brought on a very strong frustration that came out in fits of raising my voice so that I would be heard and listened to.

Then there were the mood swings. Some experts may say that a person can control their mood and the swings that come from it with a little professional help. I say that humans will always have mood swings and nothing will stop them or cure them. I have awakened in the best of moods and carried on with my daily work with a high that I do not think will be destroyed. But it takes just one small word or action and that utopia comes crashing down. In fact, it happened just the other day. My beautiful new book, so fresh and clean and hopefully perfect after having three editors and myself go over it I do not know how many times, was criticized by a very caring person who was only trying to help me further my writing career for the next book by pointing out that there were quite a few errors. The book is out, for better or for worse, and cannot be fixed now, but that feeling of accomplishment, that euphoria is gone. Do not take me wrong, for I still pat myself on the back every time I sell a book and beam from ear to ear every time someone says that they love the book, but the bright edge is gone.

All the times when I was in school, it does not matter if it was grade school, high school, or university because it happened throughout my learning. It saw all those horrible circled words mostly in red covering so many of the pages of my papers or book, the feeling that I had failed again would come over me and I would just cry. But I do believe these mishaps also made me stronger.

What do I mean by mishaps? They are problems that at the time felt very big and against me personally. I do not know to this day if they were deliberate or could have been prevented. The best way to tell you about these problematic failures is communicating it to you in a story.

It was 1986 and I was living in Hawaii, working for a man who I believe now did not know how to communicate fully what he was thinking and often his actions resulted in a calamity. Getting the position through a temporary company, and it could have gone into a permanent job, if the trouble that ended our working together was not over a paycheck.

You see, at that time in my life I was living on a shoestring and whenever money was a little freer I would not cash my check right away but lived on what I had stashed away. Knowing if the cash was there it would have been spent on something I could have done without. The mishap happened shortly after I received—as it turned out—my last check, but I am getting ahead of myself. Being a person who pays something on all of her bills each month so everyone is happy and do not get slips that say "Non-Sufficient Funds." Well, because I did not deposit my check right away but waited a week, I overdrew my checking account and got a NSF and a ten-dollar charge on top of it.

It happened on a weekend that I got the notice and promptly on Monday morning I went in to the bank see what happened. It turned out that my boss had closed his accounts with his bank and had taken all the money not waiting to see if all the outstanding checks had cleared. Mine did not. Upon reaching the office, I went straight in to see him to let him know the circumstance and the first thing out of his mouth was, "Well why didn't you cash the check?"

Even at that time in my life I knew enough to speak up for myself when realizing he was putting the blame on me. I got angry to the point that I spoke right back.

"Do you always close your accounts and not leave enough cash in the account for all checks too clear? Because there were no funds in your old account I was charged a ten-dollar NSF and I would like a replacement check and the ten dollars back."

I will paraphrase here, he said, "I will give you another check but will not pay for the NSF. And I think you really need to seek help for your temper and I do not need your assistance anymore."

To which I said, "I do not think I need any help but I think you should go and get a course on how to deal with banking needs. How many other people had trouble with your account closing?"

After leaving I went to the temporary job agency and told them what had happened and got another position. I am not sure if they dealt with him again.

Then, at the age of sixty I finally learned how to read people and understand what they were looking for and how I could get what was needed even if I did not have the confidence that I could do the job. I also know that I got to an age that I got defiant and did and said what needed to be said and in doing this found my voice.

Let me give you another example: My last position was working in a high school with Special Education students for ten years. I was mostly for the students' rights and tried to make sure that their voice was heard the best I could. One of the tasks that the students and I did was delivering the daily newspaper to all the classrooms and teachers that signed up for delivery.

Now, a student tradition that I think is finally fading but was a rite of passage for a small number of male students who walked around with their pants slung around their hips allowing for a bright pair of undergarments to show. (I do not know for sure but I believe this bright garment was just for show) and the proper garment was still in place and covered.

On this particular day helping a few of my students making the deliveries I was absent from a few of my male students who were having an encounter with one of the teachers. Coming out of their classroom, she told one of the boys to pull up his pants. When I returned from helping with the delivery there the teacher was at him again and I asked what was going on. The teacher said that "He," pointing to the student, *I am paraphrasing here* "Was told to pull up his pants and look where they are now." I asked my student if he had pulled up his pants and he said, "Yes." Returning my gaze to the teacher I got the question, "Are you taking his word over mine?"

"Yes," I said, "for as you can see he has no belt and the pants are bound to fall down again. What do you want him to do?" I asked.

The teacher returned to the classroom and promptly turned me in to the assistant principal for lack of cooperation. I was called down to the office and treated like a common criminal. This had happened to me before so it was nothing new and I usually stood up for the student. I was asked to explain and after stating what the teacher had said, I also replied that they, the teacher, had a dirty mind, for there was nothing wrong with the student's clothing that a belt could have helped.

I was asked to apologize to the teacher and refused unless there was an apology issued to the student, who was not allowed to deliver the newspaper again.

CHAPTER TEN

LIVING ALONE VS. BEING ALONE

Have you ever felt isolated and do not know how long you have felt this way? Being dyslexic can put you in this situation. My siblings and cousins were my nucleus and we were always busy it seemed. I did have one or two friends that are friends to this day and by the time I was in the second grade that seemed enough. The feelings got stronger as I entered the third grade for I did not mind playing by myself and did not realize or feel the need to reach out, to join in with the rest of the kids, unless the games or activities interested me. But by the fourth grade I was feeling that I was not quite as alert as the rest of the students. There was something wrong that made it hard for me to read. I have no recollection of being alone or lonely until the sixth to eighth grades when my differences were a lot more pronounced. This is when the ugliness and the mistreatment started and my self-preservation kicked in and to stop the hurt I closed myself off from making too many friends or joining different activities. But you must remember that I was having too hard a time just keeping up with schoolwork, especially in high school. Getting involved in extra activities or working would probably have been a disaster

My mother trying to help told me to look for someone who looked alone or lonely and go up to him or her and start talking.

So, I did see a girl one day in high school that looked alone and I did talk to her. That lasted about five minutes. She barely responded to my questions and I could tell that she was not on my wavelength of intelligence. Was that how the other students saw me? To my surprise, many times later while working in my chosen fields someone would approach me and say they remembered me from high school. So, I must have been noticed and found interesting without even realizing it even though I did not remember them.

This brings me to the question of living alone versus being alone and what is the difference? I think that people can get used to being and living alone and like it. There is a feeling of freedom when you are able to choose what you want to do and when. Living most of my life with someone that I could do something with if I felt like it, but most of the time I did not. Maybe I did not want to bother. Was I in isolation or was it that I could entertain myself better?

When I was in VISTA stationed with two very nice women that were a lot younger I was not lonely even though they tried to include me in their fun. They would drive by and ask me to join them in the car just to cruise around the small town of two thousand people and see what was happening. This for sure did not catch my interest. They were in a different place in their lives than I was, and even though we were all single, they were looking for someone to be with while I was not. Was I lonely? No, but I was alone a lot.

The same thing happened in Hawaii living by myself. The first year I had too many people around me while living at the YWCA. Then I moved out and got my own apartment by myself and later had a roommate for I wanted company when I needed it. It is not that we saw each other a lot, for she was an out-and-about person and had a male friend for company, but when she was there it was nice having her to be with.

This is where I believe being alone comes in. I want to share the things that I have seen and did in any particular day with someone at the end of the day, and there is no one. Having someone to be in the same area as I am, think on the same wavelength but not in my space all the time. Just to know that someone is there who would be willing to listen to my thoughts and have a comment about them, good or bad. There were many times when I was traveling that I would end up in a hotel room by myself at the end of the day and wish that there was someone to talk the day over with. I am sure there are many people who have felt the same way and it is not uncommon when you are dyslexic but is that loneliness or being alone when you want to be?

* * *

In my condominium I have a wonderful view from the fifteenth floor and because of the way the building is shaped I can see the airplanes coming and going from the airport that is off in the distance. Late at night, between 12:00 a.m.

and 2:00 a.m., I watch the planes coming in and wait until they land. To me this is very calming to know that the people on the plane are safe for another day and on the ground. Once in a while I would just like someone there to watch with me and maybe comment on what they are thinking as they see the planes land.

I would love to be married in this period of my life. I will turn seventy years young very soon and would really like to have someone around to share with. But when I mention this to my family and acquaintances they seem shocked or think I am crazy. I know that living with someone now after being single all my life would take a lot of adjustment on both people's parts.

But I really think it would be worth it and it is just not happening. I was told that I have to get out more and be where men are, and that is partially true. I have connected three times with men that I could have lived with in my life but marriage was not to be had. I was engaged to a real nice man seventeen year older than I who was forty-four. We had six wonderful months together, *before the Lord decided he wanted him*, and he died of a heart attack. The time was not right or maybe I was not right. The self-preservation in being different could have held me back from some commitments, but not because of the lack of courage.

Though alone, I did not feel lonely all these years and most of the time I enjoyed the feeling of being free.

CHAPTER ELEVEN

BUTTERFLY

A lot changed in 2013, some good and some sad. I retired and finished my first book called the "Dark Side Of Key West." My mother, after catching pneumonia and an a unrelated infection, landed in the hospital and then in a nursing home and I found I was on my own for the first time in sixty-six years. Not that I never lived on my own for I did three times and was always totally in charge of my affairs and chose to return to Minnesota where my heart lived. This was different.

Whenever I was in the bosom of my family there was the feeling of being sheltered and overly protected. Whenever I tried stating an opinion of my own it was shot down or not given much thought. Then I would get very frustrated and lose the little control that I had and start raising my voice for my own rights to be heard and be understood. I did not have the capacity or knowledge to fight against the onslaught of them all. I do not think my family even knew how they were lowering my self-esteem at those times and it was partially my fault for letting them do it, but I did not know how to prevent it either.

Being told that I was always wrong from a very early age made me shut down and retreat into myself with no confidence in anything that I said. The only time I felt confident was when I was out on my own and this is one of the reasons that I travel by myself. For here is where I found that people, strangers, were listening and enjoying what I was saying. I was a butterfly flying free. These were my growth periods but they only lasted for very short times when traveling.

Then, after my mother left for the nursing home, I found that I was on my own and totally in charge for my livelihood—retired, living on a fixed income, paying an association fee for a place of my own, and finally making the decisions that no one could change but me. I love my family and would not want any of them to change because they are who they are, but I am the butterfly.

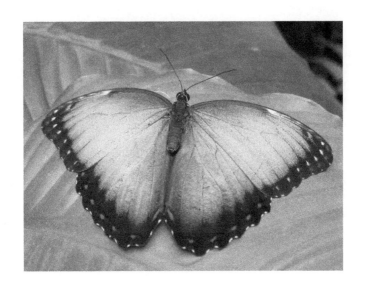

CHAPTER TWELVE

LEARNED TRICKS AND TECHNIQUES

Things that helped me during learning and still are helping: breaking up the amount of work that is needed so that it did not get discouraging, had line markers so that eyes did not skip a line when reading, finding a quiet space to read or think so no visual distraction took my attention, *the eyes are my first form of attack and my curiosity,* sat up front in most of the classrooms so I could hear and see what was be taught.

Math problems, can you imagine adding up a column in a test and hoping that there will not be a 9 or a 6 in the problem. To this day 9 and 6 are reversed every single time in math problems I have. The only good thing now is that my brain corrects itself immediately, so I can get the problem right. Practice, Practice is what it takes.

Motor problems, not wanting to play any sports in the gym for I knew that I would be the last chosen. My coordination was so bad that I still to this day walk into walls if I am not careful.

But, some positive things I have learned from working 10 years in the public-school system in Special Ed. is that dyslexics most likely have good temperaments, their outlook on life is infectious and outside of academic they have skills that they use and enjoy to the better of others.

Multisensory Approach to Learning:

Reading:

The dual-route theory of reading aloud was first described in the early 1970s. This theory suggests that two separate mental mechanisms, or cognitive routes, are involved in <u>reading</u> aloud, with output of both mechanisms contributing to the <u>pronunciation</u> of a written stimulus.

From Wikipedia, the free encyclopedia

The best practice that I have ever done for myself is to read aloud. Ever since I started reading for pleasure I have read aloud. I found out quickly that my eyes and brain do constantly get confused when I am reading. (1) That my eyes skip lines and (2) that what the eye and brain have read not always makes sense. Then I have to read the sentence or paragraph some time *over* before it sinks in and I comprehend what I had read. Reading aloud gains confidence, train yourself to look at one word at a time especially the big words. Try to move your eyes smoothly over the line which will help start a reading rhythm and this helps the brain remember what you have read.

The best books that I have read over the years are the ones that through their words the authors have given me wonderful pictures of what they are describing. Like the inside of a murder scene when the lead detective goes over the smells, position of the body, destruction of the room, blood splashing if there is any. These kinds of items being described brings the scene into play for me. That's good reading.

Use scents and color: When you mind is restless especially at stress time the scents of Lavender and vanilla help promote relaxation, Citrus, peppermint and pine help increase alertness and Cinnamon helps to improve focus. Also, the color of green, which helps increase concentration and feelings of emotional well-being, in reading areas and computer stations.

✳ ✳ ✳

As I have stated spelling incorrectly always invades my work pages. It was suggested that I get an application on my computer that would allow me to speak into a microphone and the computer program would type for me. But you must remember that you still have to say which word you are using when two words have similar or different meanings but sound alike; There and Their, Sun and Son, See and Sea the existing technology of today can help immensely in which I did not have the pleasure of using then.

Spelling:

In learning to spell I had to learn each and every word by rote. This means that if you picked up a pencil which you probably knew what it was by the time you were three. But did you know how it was spelled. No. so someone, most likely a teacher or parent would write down on a blackboard or paper the word *pencil*.

Math:

My math area of learning is just general. According to the physiologist remarks it was believed that I had reached my area of learning on the subject and she was surprised that I understood some of the beginning concepts of algebra.

In my tutoring since I retired I have help with math and reading. Math was always a difficult subject for me for I saw number mix-up and it still carries on and always will.

Numbers such as a nine for a six or 6 for a 9. Every time as a kid when I did a math problem with these two numbers I would get the problem wrong. Even though it was frustrating and made me feel stupid, the worst part was that I did not know it was those two numbers that were causing the problem. I found this out much later in life

The wonderful thing is that my brain has learned to see the numbers that cause me trouble seconds after I have put them down or spoken them wrong. There are many number that can cause trouble with dyslexic's and 12 or 21 are just two. What if you are adding a column and the above two number always get mixed up? Most dyslexics have strong visual and vivid reasoning which helps them understand math concepts, but do not realize that they are reversing numbers in their brain and the reversal can cause them trouble the rest of their life.

Let us say that they are going for a 12 not a 21 and the question is how may groups of three is there in twelve? A visual trick is to have them use an item that they can count with: like buttons or beads to count into groups of threes and see how many groups make up 12.

Note: I do take care of all my own finances but have to check often.

Organization:

Learning early that I had to have my thoughts and materials organized was a great help and most important when items are not put in order in the work place, home or car can lead to a disaster and possibly a lot more work and frustration are not far behind.

The brain is the first place to start for after a word is learned it is there but may take a few extra minutes to process. Wanting to state or relate something you think important to others, let yourself have several seconds to formulate the words. This can be frustrating but letting a minute or so pass before using a different approach can clear the brain and help your thought proceed.

Multisensory approach to learning:

This approach to learning refers to a design from the 1930's by Samuel Orton and Anna Gillingham, who wish to help dyslexic children learn to use sequential structured techniques such as:

Learn through *visual/seeing* the object or subject on a screen, computer, through a microscope, these items can clarify what the subject is saying.

Auditory/hearing:

A difficulty of understand what is said orally. This can lead to not being able to simply hear directions that are stated to them. The person can hear what is being said but the brain has a hard time listening and comprehending which can lower their performance in learning. Which can lead to problems with spelling, comprehension and reading.

This can be helped by using a tape recorder so that the information can be played back several times if necessary.

Getting the directions to work subjects clarified. Have them repeated in a different way and allow asking questions until they are understood. *(especially in a testing area.)* And one of the most important to me is the eliminating of distractions. *(like being given a quiet room when the thinking process is fully needed.)* Any little distraction such as a cough, dropping of a pencil, opening and closing to a door will take the attention away from what is most important.

Using both oral and visual presentation in teaching methods.

Last is the <u>Kinesthetic/Seeing</u>: This is where I believe I am the strongest. I have to feel and touch everything, I found that was the best way to learn. Just picking up and investigating help my understanding what the brain might be scrambling at the moment.

CHAPTER THIRTEEN

INSPIRATION

I have thought many times in the past half-decade where the power to write my first book came from and now this one. I now realize that the inspiration started in my last year of university. I wrote two papers that my professors asked me for permission to copy and use without my name, *being used*, for their future classes. I am enclosing one of the papers in the appendix for you the readers with Dyslexia--**mostly**--to show that we can be just as intelligent and inspired persons even with a brain disorder.

* * *

In my Catholic faith, we have a quiet place and time where a person can go and pray for as long as they like but an hour is a preferred amount of time given in adoration. Now it was getting to the end of my week and for my class on Taxonomy I had a paper due the next night and I had maybe a paragraph written. I knew that I needed some inspiration and where better that in my adoration hour of thought, prayer and yes to writing my paper.

The below paper is what came out of that hour and into the history of my professor's future classes as a sample of what a paper for her subject on Taxonomy can look like.

HERE IS PROOF THAT A DYSLEXIC BRAIN CAN CHANGE.

TAXONOMY OF TEACHING

The six levels of Bloom's Taxonomy have given me a good reflective introduction into urban teaching. The levels are Knowledge, Comprehension, Application, Analysis, Synthesis and Evaluation. I have chosen three to elaborate on, *knowledge, comprehension* and *evaluation* for, they show me how teachers and students can educate and learn together.

KNOWLEDGE requires a person to recognize or remember facts just as they were learned when the subject was first presented. Knowledge questions asked to students like what is the capital of Washington, who is the Secretary of the Treasury or who wrote the Scarlet Letter are known as memorized facts? These facts are building a bank of knowledge that helps us throughout our daily lives and to function in our society. Our society deals with many memorized rules every day such as driving requirements! Or currency exchange. However, does this knowledge relate well in our schools? The research done over the years shows that the lower income students when given knowledge questions can deal with excellent answers as well as someone from a higher economic background. This gives all students a higher success rating and a stronger feeling of achievement. The drawbacks are the over use of the questions given by teachers in the classroom or during test. I know that a lot of the memorized questions over the years have been long forgotten. It takes, I realize, a certain interest, love or need of the subject to retain special knowledge.

COMPREHENSION is recalling information heard or read and relating it in your own words. An example of a comprehensive question would be what is the main idea in the writing of the Constitution? Describe in your own words what makes an airplane fly? Students can answer this kind of question only if they have received the information beforehand.

These kinds of questions help students interpret, understand, demonstrate and organize their feelings in sentences, about a topic already taught. Comprehension is the ultimate purpose of reading and if a student does not understand what he/she has read they cannot go beyond the first phase of information, which is knowledge of memorization.

EVALUATION is a judgment of a higher-order of mental process. The students learn the merit of their ideas, the power of a solution to a problem, and their opinion. To evaluate they learn to understand, reflect, choose and compare their answers to any question.

The following are some examples of Evaluation questions. How do you assess your performance at school, which U.S. Congressman is the most effective and why? When giving their opinion on the judgment or merits of an issue, the students are using their personal set of values to make the evaluation.

An evaluation can also be objective and this is taking the merit of an issue or criteria and judging the problem to an attentive solution. The important thing to remember is that Evaluation questions are judgments and can have different possible answers.

In conclusion, "In 1956 Benjamin Bloom and his team of educators developed a classification of levels of intellectual behavior important in learning, this became Taxonomy..."

> (Internet MCQs and Bloom's Taxonomy, MegaSpider.com 1998)

One might ask why Bloom wrote these objectives and how do they fit into urban teaching and effective learning? We want the students to be able to memorize (*Knowledge*) *the* basis-laws, issues and standards that are required by society. To read for the sheer joy of it and to understand *(Comprehension)* what they read. Also, to be able to appraise, compare, defend and judge the situations that life is going to place before them *(Evaluation)*. This I feel would be effective teaching and a good use of Bloom's Taxonomy.

> Essays written by: Randymary de Rosier while at Metropolitan State University. October 11, 2001,

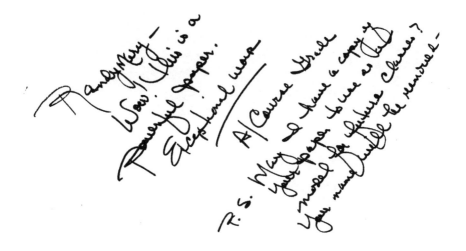

Randy/Mary -
Wow! This is a
Powerful paper.
Exceptional work.

P.S. May I have a copy of
your paper to use as (the)
model for future classes?
Your name will be removed -

A/Course Grade

CHAPTER FOURTEEN

CONCLUSION

In France, it was proven that schools that taught with phonics produced less dyslexic students than schools that taught with whole word methods. However, the true sight-word method was generally discredited in Europe by the 1970's. Change was brought about by such things as those reported in a 1950 article in France, which stated that 2% of dyslexic children, were discovered in schools, that used the phonics approach, learned faster than 20% of dyslexic children that used the sight-word method which I was taught. **www.facebook.com/public/Geraldine-Rodgers**

There are many different programs that I read about that children were taught. For instance, the letter sounds. Usually it was done in the simplest possible mechanical way. For example, the child was taught the consonant sound like drilled on the consonant-vowel combinations arranged in column form, such ba, be, bi, bo, bu; da, de, di, do, du etc. the purpose of the drill was to develop the hearing and sight enabling the child to develop as quickly as possible an automatic association between letter and sound and learning to read the alphabetic writing system.

Going Backwards

There was one program that was thought better for children to look at whole words as pictures and have them associate them directly with objects, actions and ideas rather than have them learn to associate the letters with sounds. And this is the way that I learned how to read. This I believe is part of the alphabetic learning process but I am still not sure how I learned words like: **the, an, or, but, how**, where there are not pictures to relate to even though these words can be considered connection words.

Essentially, the method works as follows: the child is given a sight vocabulary to memorize. He is taught to look and say the word without knowing that the letters stand for sounds. As far as the pupil is concerned, the letters are a bunch of arbitrary squiggles arranged in some arbitrary, haphazard order. His task is to see a picture in the configuration of the whole word – to make the word horse look like a horse.

Smart But Feeling Dumb,

It is estimated that many million dyslexic Americans have symptoms as follows: (1) memory instability for letters, words, or numbers; (2) a tendency to skip over or scramble letters, words, and sentences; (3) poor, slow, fatiguing reading ability prone to compensatory head tilting, near-far focusing, and finger pointing; (4) reversal of letters such as *b, d*, words such as *saw* and *was*, and numbers such as 6 and 9 or 16 and 61. Most of these symptoms sound like the 1912 way of learning by a sight vocabulary and also ring a bell with me.

Types of Reading Disorders (Share internet)

Dyslexia is a brain-based type of learning disability that specifically impairs a person's ability to read. Individuals with dyslexia typically read at levels significantly lower than expected despite having normal intelligence. Although the disorder varies from person to person, common characteristics among people with dyslexia are difficulty with phonological processing (the manipulation of sounds), spelling, and/or rapid visual-verbal responding. Dyslexia can be inherited in some families, and recent studies have identified a number of genes that may predispose an individual to developing dyslexia. Examples of specific types of reading disorders include:

- **Word decoding.** People who have difficulty sounding out written words; matching the letters to sounds to be able to read a word.
- **Lack of fluency.** People who lack fluency have difficulty reading quickly, accurately, and with proper expression (if reading aloud).
- **Poor reading comprehension.** People with poor reading comprehension have trouble understanding what they read.
- **NIH- Eunice Kennedy Shriver, National Institute of Child Health and Human Development**

Dyslexia Affects Hearing Process

Left Brain Activity Differs from Nonimpaired Readers and is helped by all the senses.

Listening

From the WebMD Archives, Oct. 27, 2003

It is becoming increasingly evident that people with dyslexia process sound and language differently from people who don't have trouble reading. Using a highly precise imaging technique, University of Texas researchers compared brain activity in areas known to be associated with analyzing the sound structure of written and spoken words in children with dyslexia with children without reading problems.

They found that the areas of the left-brain associated with speech were highly active in the nonimpaired readers and not very active at all in those who were dyslexic.

The findings are consistent with the idea that problems understanding the "sound structure" of both written and spoken language are associated with abnormal activity in this area of the brain, the researchers say.

"We are not the only ones to find that this neurological deficit appears to be confined to very restricted areas of the brain," Researcher Joshua Breier, PhD, tells WebMD. "The evidence is overwhelming that dyslexia is a very specific learning disability, and not a problem with intellect."

What if you were the one out of ten whose brain did not live up to its national intelligence and you were diagnosed with Dyslexia? Would you be willing to work ten time harder than most other people to get what you wanted to use your brain for the common good of the World?

We have/had many people who did just that and were dyslexic. People like: John F. Kennedy- president, Tom Cruise- actor, Whoopi Goldberg-actress, Albert Einstein-Theoretical physicist-genius, Jeremy Bonderman-baseball major league, Muhammad Ali. boxer, Patrick Dempsey-race car driver, Charles Conrad Jr.-Astronaut and Leonardo de Vinci – inventor.

In the 1950 the U.S. was reporting that it has children whose intellectual abilities were as normal as any other child without this brain disorder, but they could not read, write, or spell correctly. This malfunction of the brain can cause if not caught and helped with training: 1. Difficulty in academic achievement, 2. lack of success in employment, 3. If employed difficulty with keeping a job because of a slower functioning brain, trouble with remember numbers and names, 4. Which causes the reduction of self-confidence and esteem. Even with help the dyslexic well struggle with reading and writing all their life but will be creative people filling many important positions in our world by navigating a different path but still contributing by fulfilling successful lives.

POST SCRIPT

The above paper which I wrote for one of my Education classes on Taxonomy of Teaching gave me a wonderful surprise. Besides getting an "A" in my class I was also given a wonderful gift. The professor of my class asked me for a copy of my paper, for their future classes.

Readers, this does happen to people with Dyslexia right along with any other students in university. The only thing is not so often and we just have to keep going and learning with life as much as we can to keep our spirits high.

Thanks for reading and keep learning,

Randymary de Rosier

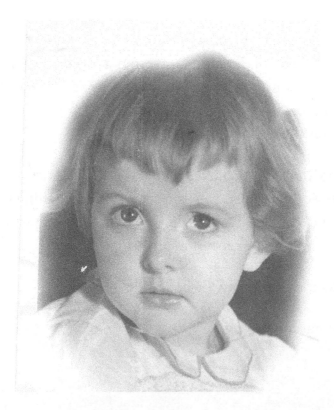

Randy at 2 taken by her father who was also Dyslexic.

Lightning Source UK Ltd.
Milton Keynes UK
UKHW010618100223
416791UK00001B/12